SO-AZU-362

My Hometown
Mashpee

Story by Barbara Gleason

Illustrated by Emma Eichner

Get out and explore!
- Barbara Gleason

AuthorHouse™
1663 Liberty Drive
Bloomington, IN 47403
www.authorhouse.com
Phone: 1-800-839-8640

© 2009 Barbara Gleason, Illustrated by Emma Eichner. All rights reserved.

No part of this book may be reproduced, stored in a retrieval system, or transmitted by any means without the written permission of the author.

First published by AuthorHouse 8/18/2009

ISBN: 978-1-4389-9984-5 (SC)

Printed in the United States of America
Bloomington, Indiana

This book is printed on acid-free paper.

authorHOUSE®

For my husband, John...your continued support and unconditional love is what makes everything in my life possible.

And for my two beautiful children who have blessed me in so many ways... there isn't a day that goes by without you amazing me. You were the inspiration for this book. Thank you for teaching me.

I'm Molly from Mashpee and
I want you to know,

Some of my most favorite
places to go!

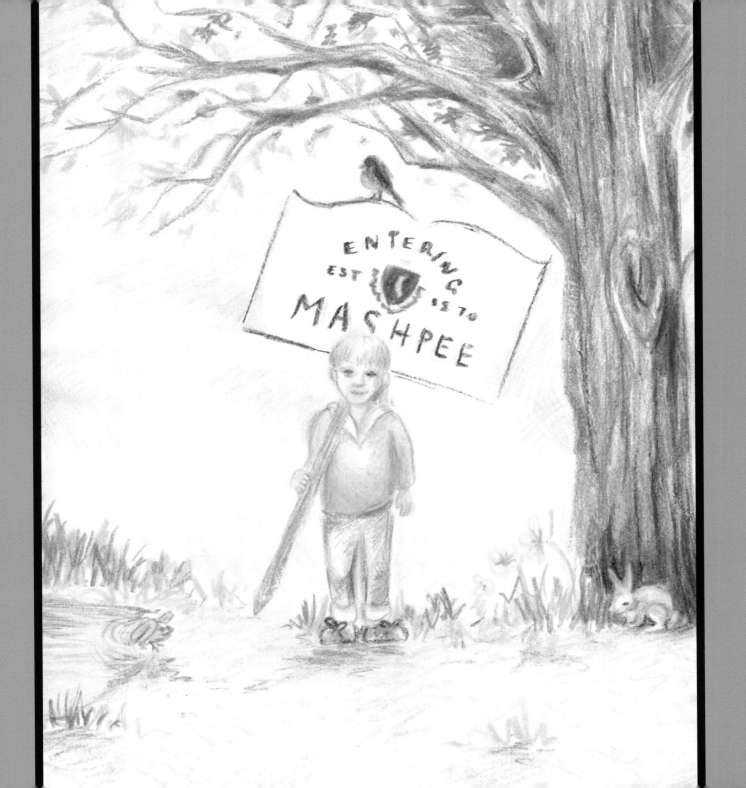

But first, I will make a
snack to bring along.

This Mashpee Munch will help
keep me healthy and strong!

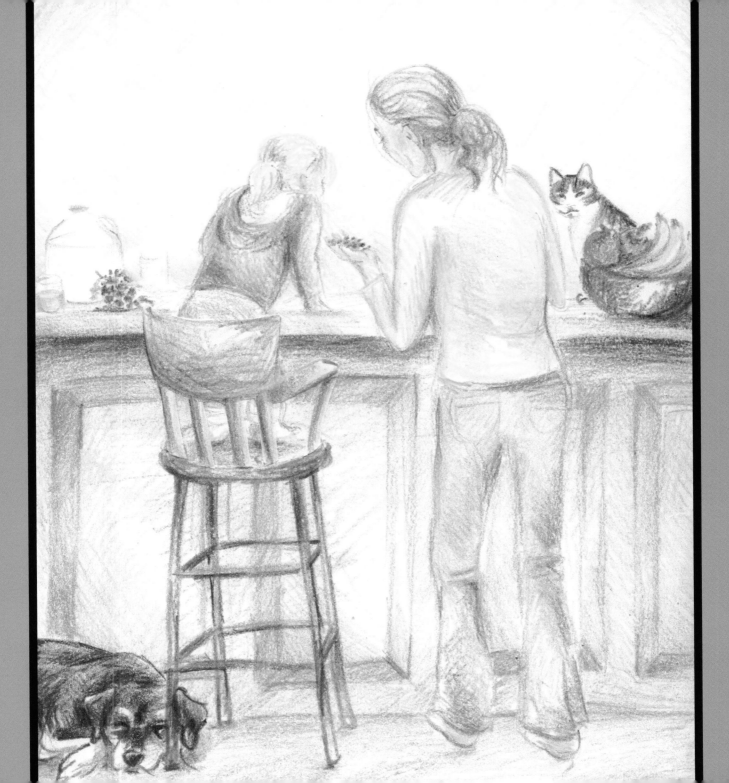

The Children's Museum is a place
to create, dream, imagine and play.

My grandparents watch me interact with
toys, puzzles and instruments all day!

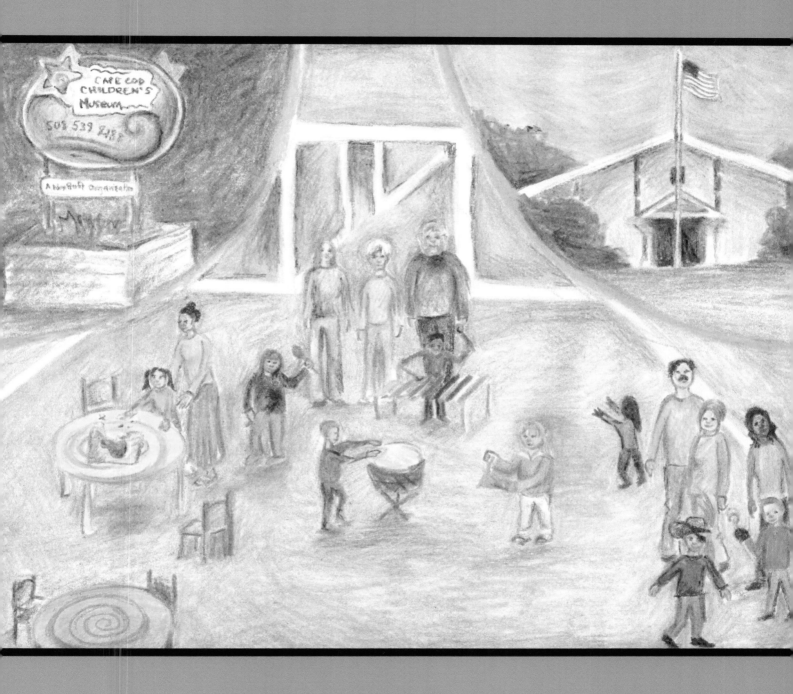

Off with Mommy and Daddy
to South Cape I go,

With balls and buckets
and shovels in tow.

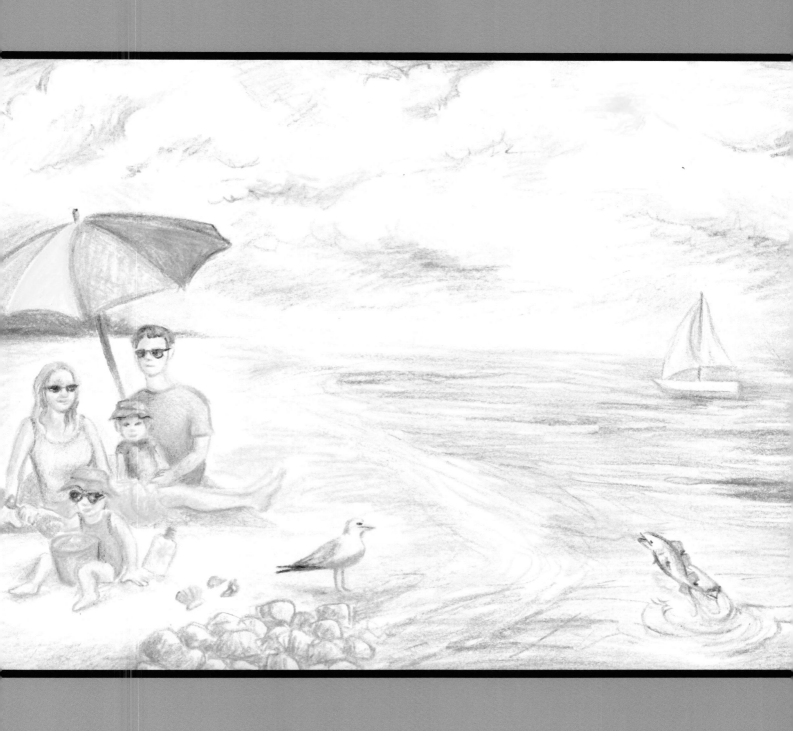

The library is always such
a fun place to be.

Here, my aunt and uncle
read with me under a tree.

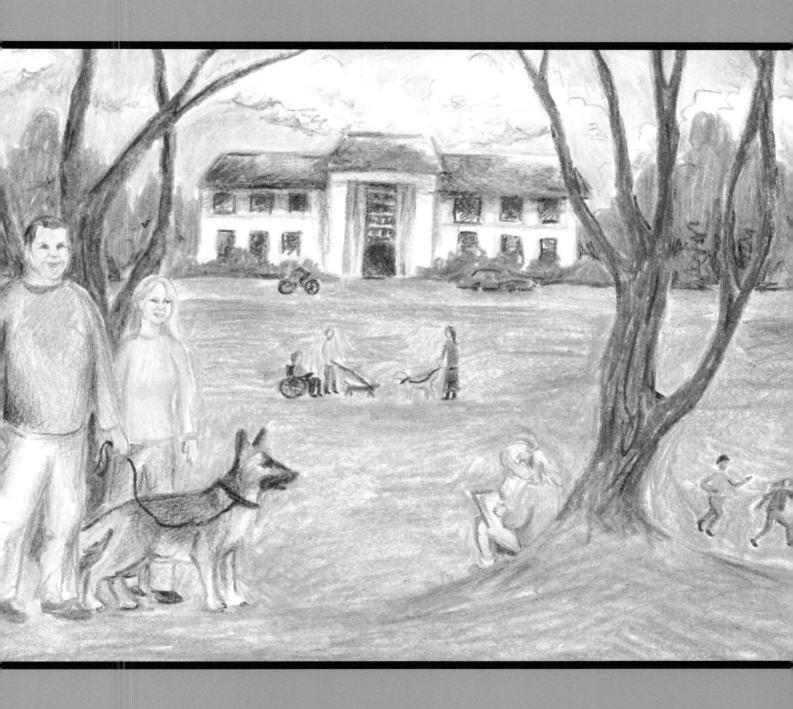

On a nice sunny day,
Mashpee Commons is grand.

Window shopping is fun while
holding Mommy's hand.

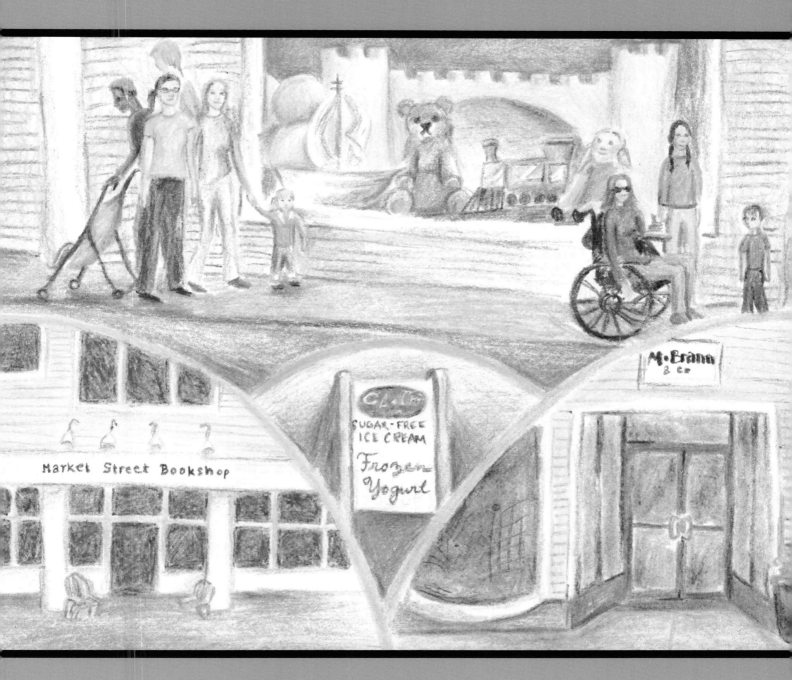

Dancing, singing and brilliant
crafts everywhere,

The Pow Wow has plenty
of culture to share.

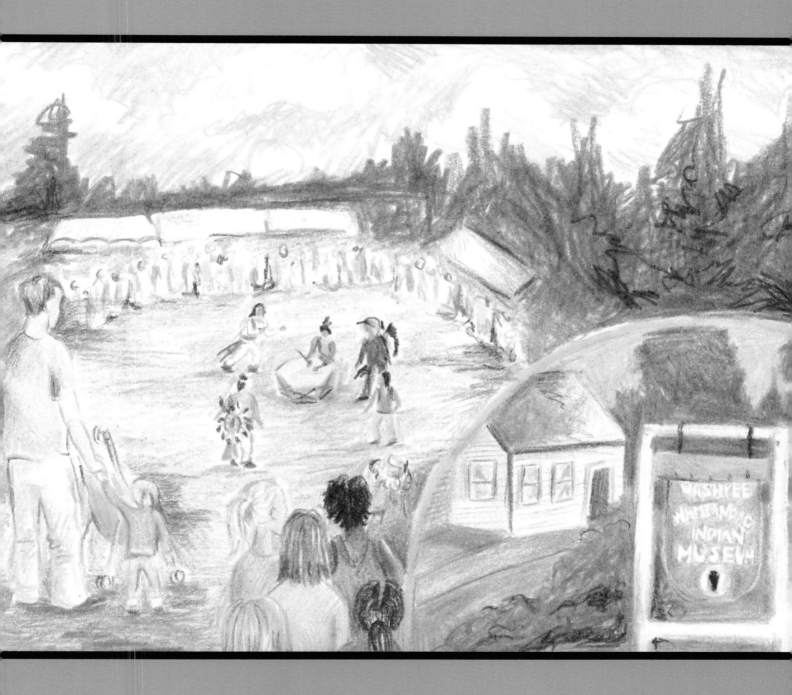

There is so much to see
in New Seabury too,

But playing mini-golf is my
favorite thing to do.

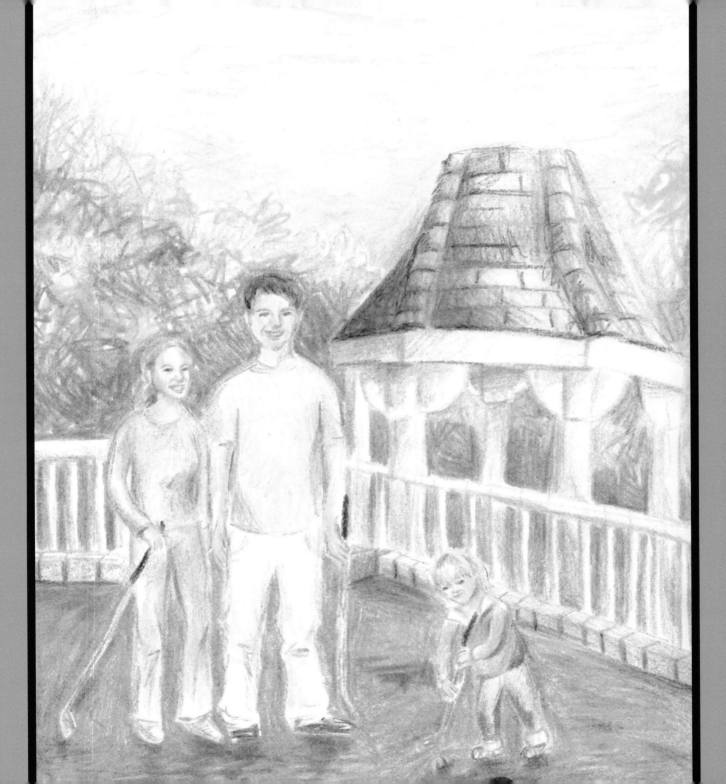

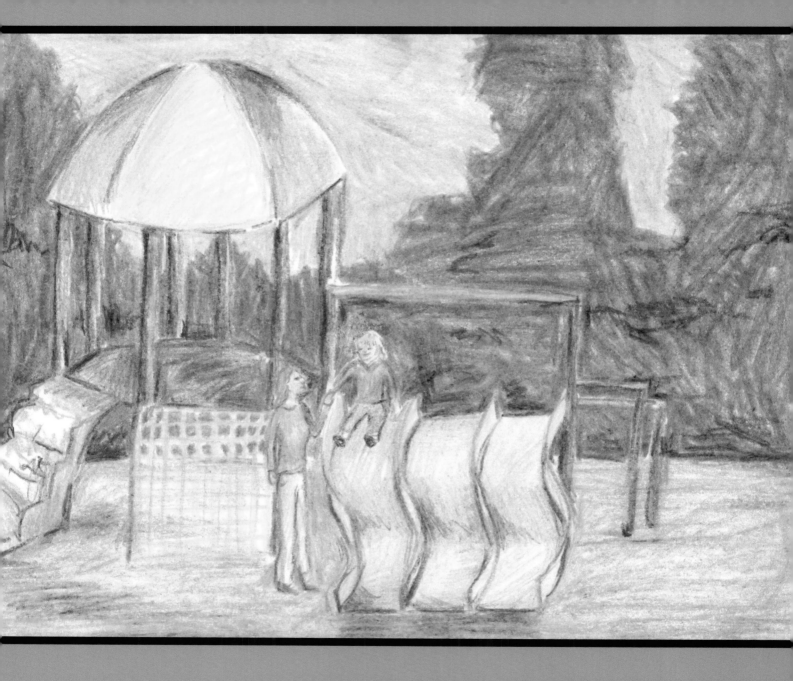

Heritage Park has the best
playground around,

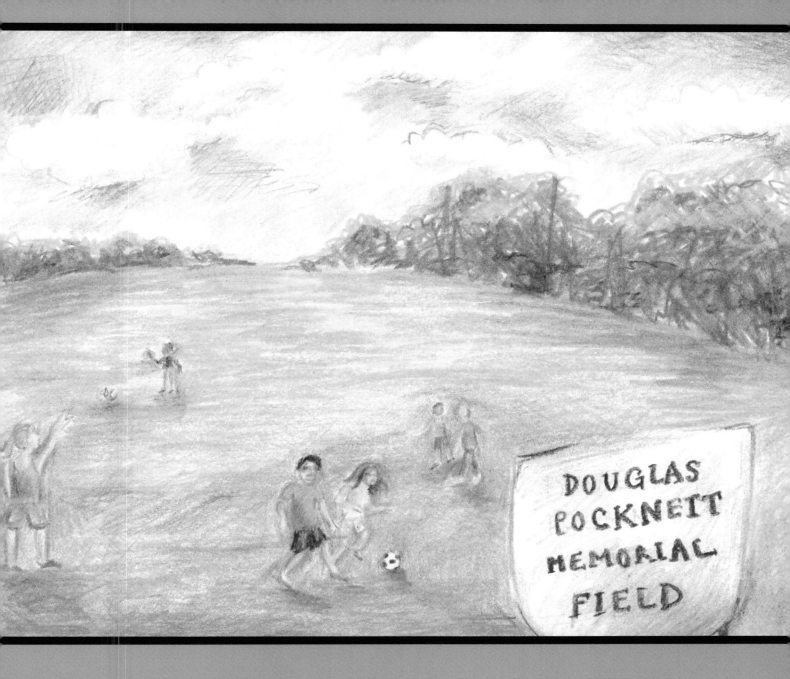

From swinging to sliding or
kicking balls on the ground.

The Woodlands is our
last stop in Mashpee,

Walking trails, seeing birds,
the river and the trees.

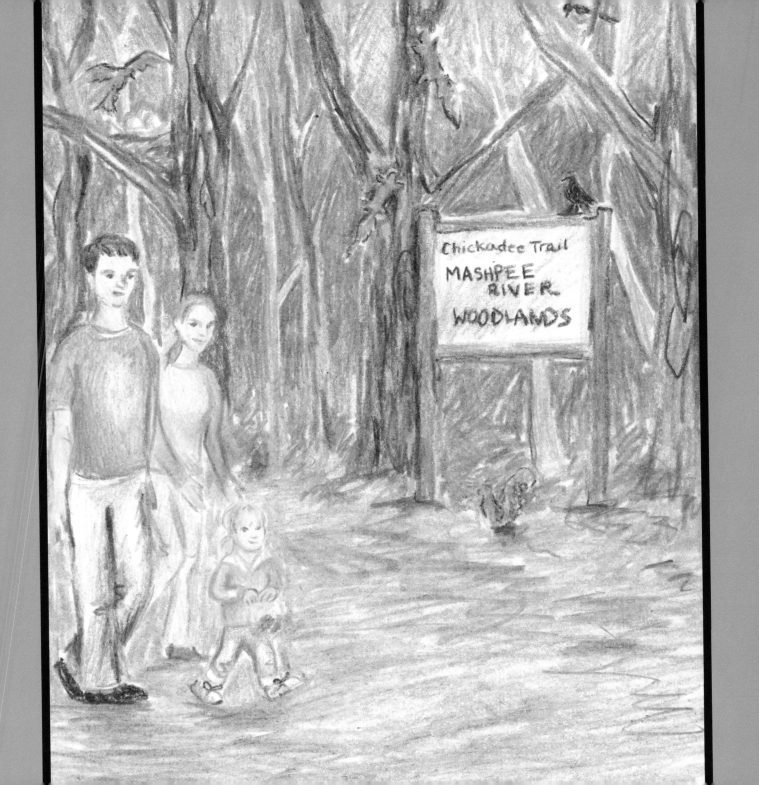

I'm glad I packed my
Mashpee Munch to eat on the way,

Because it gave me enough
energy to get through the day.

Mashpee has so many fun
things to see and do.

Maybe someday you can do
all these fun things too!

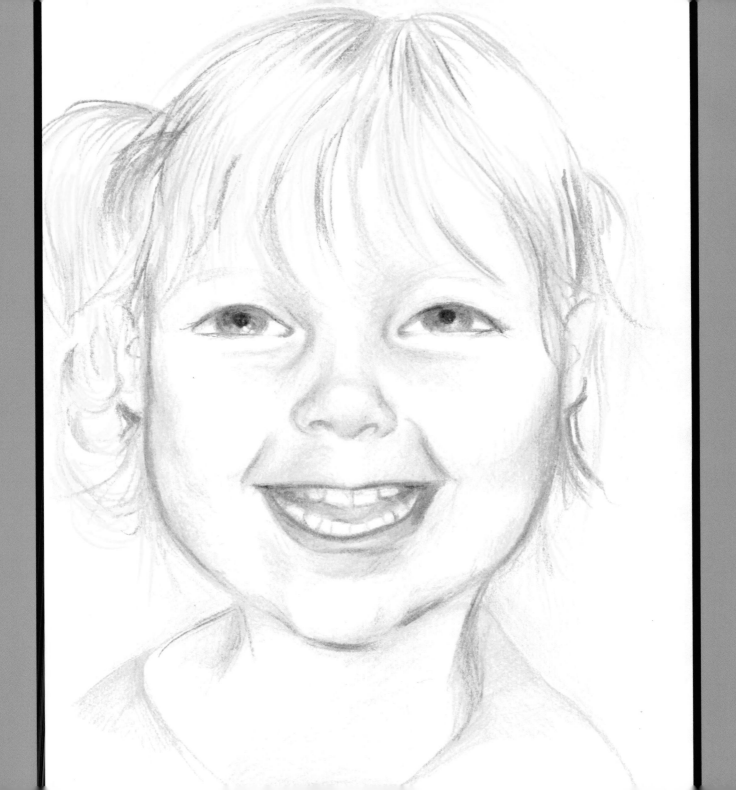

For more information:

www.myhometownbooks.com

MOLLY'S MASHPEE MUNCH

½ cup of Kashi 7-Grain Honey Cereal
½ cup of Cheddar Goldfish
½ cup of raisins
½ cup of Cherrios
½ cup of dried bananas

Feel free to substitute or add other healthy snacks as desired. Please keep in mind age requirements for food allergies and choking hazards.

LaVergne, TN USA
28 August 2009
156165LV00002BA